Natural Cosmetics

15 Homemade Organic Makeup Recipes

Table of Contents

Introduction

There you are, going through your makeup bag, and trying to decide what you want for the night. You've been looking forward to this night for a long time, and you are getting ready for the fun.

But, as you flip through what you have available, you realize that most of the ingredients are things you have been wanting to avoid. After all, you love all natural, organic ingredients because they leave you with the best results, and you don't have to worry about what they may do to your skin.

Yet it doesn't appear as though you have anything like that. You see eye shadow, lipstick, foundation powder, blemish cover up, and all kinds of other makeup, but what you don't see is anything organic.

You want to know that what you put on your skin is healthy, and there's not going to be anything wrong with it. You want to make sure there are no side effects, that you don't have to worry about wrinkles, breakouts, or clogged pores, and that you don't have to worry that what you are putting on your skin is worse than what you are covering up.

If you want to find the solution to perfect makeup, you have to go organic. Better yet, you should learn how to make it yourself, so you are in complete control of the results. But that brings up another question… how?

How are you supposed to make our own makeup? Isn't it hard? Does it last? Can you make makeup that works for what you need, and is as good as what you are used to?

The answer is exactly what you are hoping for… yes. Not only is makeup easy to make, but you can get just as good of results as you would with store bought makeup, for less money and better ingredients.

That's right. When you know how to make your own makeup, you are going to uncover the secret you need to healthy skin. No more stressing about what goes into the makeup, no more wondering if you are doing more harm than good on your skin, and no more wondering how you are going to get the makeup you want, to the standards you want.

Get ready to discover the joys of making your own makeup, and never go back to the store bought varieties again.

Let's get started.

Chapter 1 – Youthful, Perfect Skin

Everyone wants that glowing, flawless skin, but if you have ever tried to purchase foundation in the store, you know that there are countless ingredients in the powders that you can't pronounce or that you don't want to put on your face.

You want something that works, something that is all natural, and something you can have full confidence in as you spread it across your face. It can take some trial and error, but if you follow the recipes I have provided here, you are going to get the foundation you have been looking for.

I have worked on each and every one of these recipes diligently, so you can rest assured they are going to blend with your skin color, cover anything you want covered, and last all day long. Get ready to say goodbye to the cosmetics you have been spending hundreds of dollars on every year, as soon as you try any one of these recipes you will be hooked.

Practice with each recipe and find the one you like the best, then work to get the right shade, and your organic powder is going to be ready.

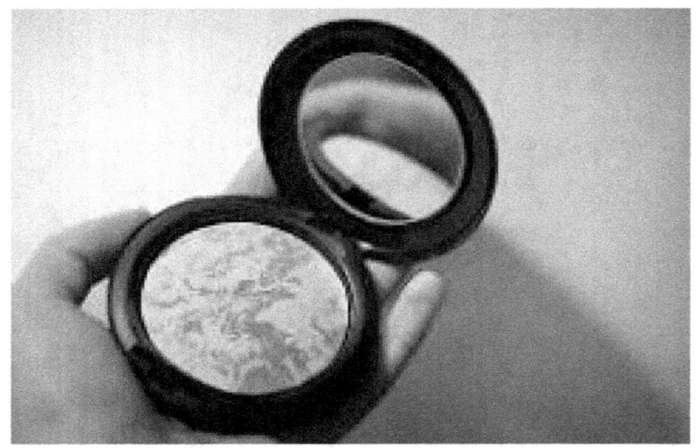

Falling in Love with Liquid

What you will need:

All natural, organic lotion

Organic Earth Clay

Organic cocoa powder

Zinc Oxide Powder

Directions:

To make this liquid foundation, you can use a blender, emulsifier, or simply mix it with a fork or whisk if you want to do the entire thing by hand.

Start with ¼ cup lotion in a bowl. This is the base of your makeup, and the rest of the ingredients you will add slowly, a little of each at a time, until you are happy with the color.

I find it best to sprinkle some of each of the powders into the lotion, then use your fork or blender to blend. Add the darker powders to darken the look, or the lighter powders to lighten.

Have a mirror handy, and use a brush or your fingers to apply a bit of the makeup to your cheeks and forehead. Keep a jar of makeup remover handy, and remove between tests.

Play around with the colors until you are happy with the look, and you are done!

Store the liquid foundation in a small, airtight jar, and shake or mix before use.

Beauty is as Beauty Does

What you will need:

Arrowroot powder

Cinnamon

Nutmeg

Coco powder

Turmeric powder

White flour

Earth Clay Powder

1 teaspoon almond oil

Directions:

You could use an emulsifier with this recipe, but I find it easiest to simply mix it all by hand. Use a large bowl, and keep an air tight jar handy to store when you are done, and you are ready to begin.

As you can see, each of the ingredients used has vastly different colors. They are all natural ingredients, and you ought to be using organic sources for all of them. The key now is to blend the ingredients together to get the color of your own skin.

Nutmeg and cinnamon are both incredibly good for your skin, so feel free to use as much of these as you like. If you want a darker foundation, start with a smaller base of arrowroot powder, but if you want a lighter foundation, start with a larger base.

Carefully mix the dry ingredients first, then finish with the oil. Make sure all is mixed and that there are no lumps.

Have a mirror handy, and use a brush or your fingers to apply a bit of the makeup to your cheeks and forehead. Keep a jar of makeup remover handy, and remove between tests... if you want a darker shade, try adding more cocoa powder. If you want lighter, use the nutmeg. It's going to be a lot of trial and error for your own particular skin type, but with a few test runs, you'll get it.

Play around with the colors until you are happy with the look, and you are done!

Store the powder in a small, airtight jar, and shake or mix before use.

Powdered Power

What you will need:

Ground nutmeg

Powdered cinnamon

Powdered cocoa powder

Bentonite clay

1 teaspoon jojoba oil

Corn starch

Directions:

You could use an emulsifier with this recipe, but I find it easiest to simply mix it all by hand. Use a large bowl, and keep an air tight jar handy to store when you are done, and you are ready to begin.

As you can see, each of the ingredients used has vastly different colors. They are all natural ingredients, and you ought to be using organic sources for all of them. The key now is to blend the ingredients together to get the color of your own skin.

Nutmeg and cinnamon are both incredibly good for your skin, so feel free to use as much of these as you like. If you want a darker foundation, start with a smaller base of arrowroot powder, but if you want a lighter foundation, start with a larger base.

Carefully mix the dry ingredients first, then finish with the oil. Make sure all is mixed and that there are no lumps.

Have a mirror handy, and use a brush or your fingers to apply a bit of the makeup to your cheeks and forehead. Keep a jar of makeup remover handy, and remove between tests.

Again, if you want a darker shade, try adding more cocoa powder. If you want lighter, use the nutmeg. It's going to be a lot of trial and error for your own particular skin type, but with a few test runs, you'll get it.

Play around with the colors until you are happy with the look, and you are done! Store the powder in a small, airtight jar, and shake or mix before use.

Chapter 2 – It's All in the Eyes

Let's face it, we are all in love with those dramatic, beautiful eyes, and we would give anything to have eyes like that every day of the week.

But, as you know, our skin absorbs so many things through the skin around the eyes, and you don't want to put anything near your eyes that can be bad for you.

With these shadows, liners, and mascaras, you can rest assured knowing that you are doing what is best for your skin while achieving the look you want.

Have fun with the colors and mix and match until you get the shade you want, then get out there and flaunt your look. There's no way you can go wrong with each of these products, so have a ball making them to be as custom as you want!

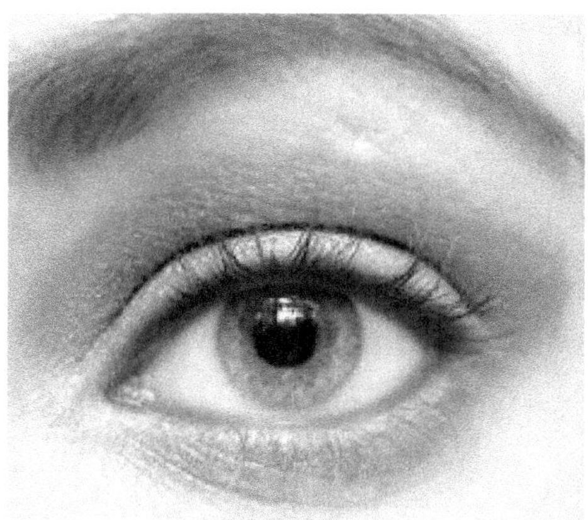

Eye Shadow for a Queen

What you will need:

Fractionated coconut oil

Eye safe mica powder

Corn starch

Directions:

You can find organic mica powder in a variety of online outlets, so shop around to find the price you like. There are going to be eye safe varieties… meaning you can use it to make eye shadow safely. Source all of your ingredients, and use a plate and a fork to blend the colors.

Carefully mix the dry ingredients first, then finish with the oil. Make sure all is mixed and that there are no lumps.

When you add the oil, you are going to add only a couple of drops at a time… this is what will make the eye shadow stay on your eyes.

Have a mirror handy, and use a brush or your fingers to apply a bit of the makeup to your eye lids. Keep a jar of makeup remover handy, and remove between tests.

Again, if you want a darker shade, try adding more mica powder. If you want lighter, add more corn starch. It's going to be a lot of trial and error for your own particular skin type and preferences, but with a few test runs you'll get it.

Play around with the colors until you are happy with the look, and you are done!

Store the powder in a small, airtight jar, and shake or mix before use.

Loving the Liner

What you will need:

Corn starch

Coconut oil

Cocoa powder

Mica powder

Activated charcoal

Directions:

You can find organic mica powder in a variety of online outlets, so shop around to find the price you like. There are going to be eye safe varieties… meaning you can use it to make eye shadow safely. Source all of your ingredients, and use a plate and a fork to blend the colors.

If you are looking for a wild or out of the ordinary color, try mica powder. If you are going to use brown or black, try using the activated charcoal or cocoa powder. You can even achieve nice colors with cinnamon, nutmeg, or turmeric.

Carefully mix the dry ingredients first, then finish with the oil. Make sure all is mixed and that there are no lumps.

When you add the oil, you are going to add only a couple of drops at a time… this is what will make the eye liner doesn't become too runny. Add enough to make it pasty, but not a full liquid.

Have a mirror handy, and use a brush or your fingers to apply a bit of the makeup to your eye lids. Keep a jar of makeup remover handy, and remove between tests.

Again, if you want a darker shade, try adding more mica powder. If you want lighter, add more corn starch. It's going to be a lot of trial and error for your own particular skin type and preferences, but with a few test runs you'll get it.

Play around with the colors until you are happy with the look, and you are done! Store the powder in a small, airtight jar, and shake or mix before use.

Mascara Madness

What you will need:

Coconut oil

Mica powder

Corn starch

Activated charcoal

Mica powder

Directions:

You can find organic mica powder in a variety of online outlets, so shop around to find the price you like. There are going to be eye safe varieties… meaning you can use it to make eye shadow safely. Source all of your ingredients, and use a plate and a fork to blend the colors.

If you are looking for a wild or out of the ordinary color, try mica powder. If you are going to use brown or black, try using the activated charcoal or cocoa powder. You can even achieve nice colors with cinnamon, nutmeg, or turmeric.

Carefully mix the dry ingredients first, then finish with the oil. Make sure all is mixed and that there are no lumps.

When you add the oil, you are going to add only a couple of drops at a time... this is what will make the mascara doesn't become too runny. Add enough to make it pasty, but not a full liquid.

Have a mirror handy, and use a brush to apply a bit of the makeup to your eye lashes. Keep a jar of makeup remover handy, and remove between tests.

Again, if you want a darker shade, try adding more mica powder. If you want lighter, add more corn starch. It's going to be a lot of trial and error for your own particular skin type and preferences, but with a few test runs you'll get it.

Play around with the colors until you are happy with the look, and you are done!

Store the powder in a small, airtight jar, and shake or mix before use.

Chapter 3 – Cherry Lipstick (For Starters)

There is just something captivating about that classic, red lipped look. But as soon as you head to the store, you see countless products that are all claiming to work, but you can't read the ingredient label.

You want something that gives you color, but you don't want to put something so close to your mouth when you aren't even sure what it is, and you don't want to spend that money on a product that you aren't entirely sold on.

When you make your own lipstick, you know exactly what it is you are getting. With these recipes, you are not only going to get the color you want, but you can add flavor and all kinds of lip-enriching ingredients.

Go ahead, have some fun, and fall in love.

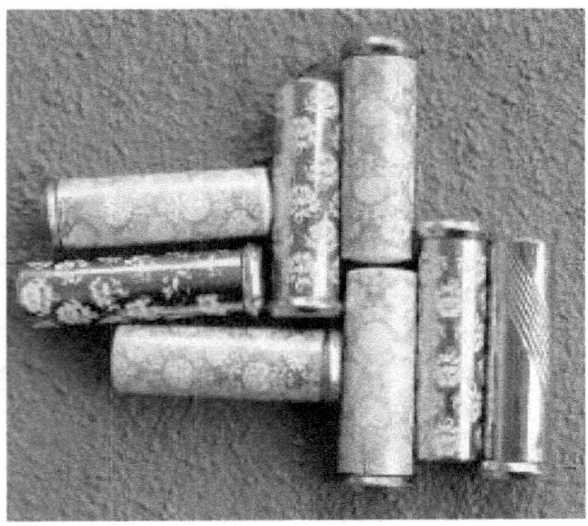

Cherry Red Lipstick

What you will need:

¼ cup beeswax

Mica powder in reds

Shea butter

1 teaspoon almond oil

Cherry essential oil

Chapstick tubes

Directions:

Using a double boiler or a pan inside a pan filled with water, add in your ¼ cup beeswax, shaved or cut into small cubes, 1/3 cup shea butter, and 1 teaspoon almond oil.

Melt these ingredients, then begin adding your mica powder. You can find mica powder in a variety of online outlets, and you can find it in a variety of colors. Find the ones you like the best, and use these.

I like deep, deep red, and to make this color, I use a combination of different shades of the powder until I find the one I like.

Once you are happy with the color, add in a few drops of the essential oil, until you have the scent you like as well. Transfer the waxy liquid to the tubes and let set up.

After they have set up for a few hours, you are ready to use!

Nude Nation

What you will need:

¼ cup beeswax

Mica powder in reds

Shea butter

1 teaspoon almond oil

Rose and peppermint essential oil

Chapstick tubes

Directions:

Using a double boiler or a pan inside a pan filled with water, add in your ¼ cup beeswax, shaved or cut into small cubes, 1/3 cup shea butter, and 1 teaspoon almond oil.

Melt these ingredients, then begin adding your mica powder. You can find mica powder in a variety of online outlets, and you can find it in a variety of colors. Find the ones you like the best, and use these.

I like my nude to still have a hue of pink to it, so when I made this lipstick, I still use some of the reds in the mica powder, just not as much. I work at it until I get the color I want, but it can take time sometimes.

Don't be afraid to work on some trial and error to get what you are after, it's worth it.

Once you are happy with the color, add in a few drops of the essential oil, until you have the scent you like as well. Transfer the waxy liquid to the tubes and let set up.

After they have set up for a few hours, you are ready to use!

Everything Lipstick

What you will need:

¼ cup beeswax

Mica powder in any color of your choice

Shea butter

1 teaspoon almond oil

Cherry essential oil

Chapstick tubes

Directions:

Using a double boiler or a pan inside a pan filled with water, add in your ¼ cup beeswax, shaved or cut into small cubes, 1/3 cup shea butter, and 1 teaspoon almond oil.

Melt these ingredients, then begin adding your mica powder. You can find mica powder in a variety of online outlets, and you can find it in a variety of colors. Find the ones you like the best, and use these.

I like deep and bold colors, so to make the colors I want, I use a combination of different shades of the powder until I find the one I like.

Once you are happy with the color, add in a few drops of the essential oil, until you have the scent you like as well. Transfer the waxy liquid to the tubes and let set up.

After they have set up for a few hours, you are ready to use!

Chapter 4 – Princess Hands

Everyone wants those pretty nails, no matter what kind of job you work. Some can have bright and elaborate nails, others have to keep theirs trim and subtle, but with these polishes, you are going to get what you want, when you want it.

Whether you are able to rock the look all throughout the week, or if you have to save your glamor for the weekend, you are going to get just what you want with each and every one of these polishes.

Have fun, throw in your own style, and get ready to walk the runway like the princess you are.

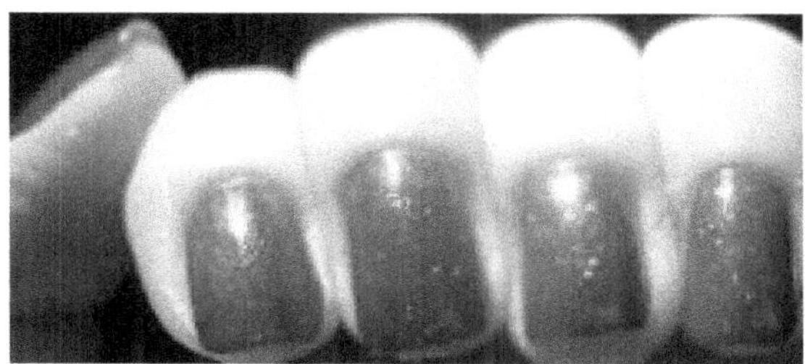

Bold and Pretty Fingernails

What you will need:

All natural, organic clear nail polish

Coconut oil

Mica powder

Glitter powder

Vitamin E oil

Airtight jar and small brush

Directions:

If your jar is large enough for you to get a stick into, I recommend you combine all the ingredients in the same jar you are going to store the polish in.

If you can't get anything in the jar, go ahead and use a small bowl or dish for mixing.

Pour all the polish into the container of choice, then sprinkle in the mica powder of your choice. Mica powder can be purchased in a variety of online outlets in virtually any color you can imagine. Add in the glitter powder, a little at a time.

You don't want to add too much, keep an eye on it until it's about the same consistency as the other polish you have used. Add in 3 drops vitamin E oil.

Mix well, and store in your airtight container.

When you are ready to use, apply 1 layer and let dry, then repeat.

Happy Heart Fingernails

What you will need:

All natural, organic clear nail polish

Coconut oil

Mica powder in reds

Airtight jar and small brush

Vitamin E oil

Directions:

If your jar is large enough for you to get a stick into, I recommend you combine all the ingredients in the same jar you are going to store the polish in.

If you can't get anything in the jar, go ahead and use a small bowl or dish for mixing.

Pour all the polish into the container of choice, then sprinkle in the mica powder of your choice. Mica powder can be purchased in a variety of online outlets in virtually any color you can imagine. Add in the colors, a little at a time until you get the shade you want.

You don't want to add too much, keep an eye on it until it's about the same consistency as the other polish you have used. Add in 3 drops vitamin E oil.

Mix well, and store in your airtight container.

When you are ready to use, apply 1 layer and let dry, then repeat.

Good For You Nail Polish

What you will need:

All natural, organic clear nail polish

Coconut oil

Vitamin E oil

Airtight jar and small brush

Directions:

If your jar is large enough for you to get a stick into, I recommend you combine all the ingredients in the same jar you are going to store the polish in.

If you can't get anything in the jar, go ahead and use a small bowl or dish for mixing.

Pour all the polish into the container of choice, then add in 6 drops of coconut oil. You can add more or less, depending on the consistency you want your polish to be. Keep in mind the thinner the polish, the harder it's going to be to apply, so add your oils slowly.

You don't want to add too much, keep an eye on it until it's about the same consistency as the other polish you have used. Add in 3 drops vitamin E oil.

Mix well, and store in your airtight container.

When you are ready to use, apply 1 layer and let dry, then repeat.

Chapter 5 – Perfectly Pampered Choices

Whether you are going with eyes, lips, or foundation, you are going to get just what you want when you are making your own makeup. But, you don't have to stop there. With this chapter, you are going to not only get blush, but hair products as well.

There's no end to the ways you can beautify and stick to your regimen, all without buying cosmetics made of artificial ingredients.

Indulge in all of the organic and natural ways you can enhance your beauty, and fall in love with the results time and time again. There's no end to the ways you can pamper yourself, so dive all in.

You deserve it.

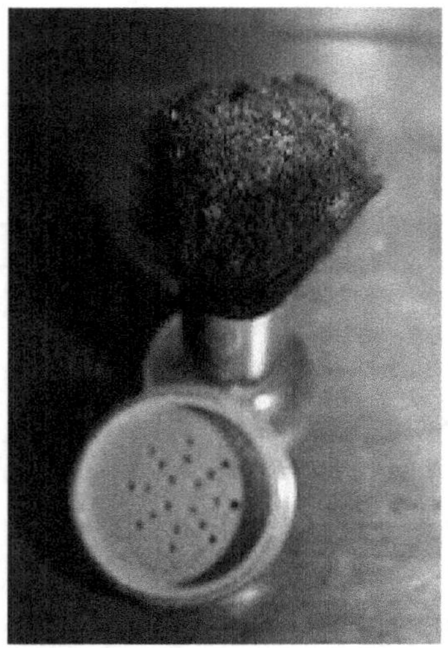

Blushing Beauty

What you will need:

Arrowroot powder

Mica powder in red

Cocoa powder

Airtight container

1 teaspoon almond oil

Directions:

Use a plate and a fork to blend the powders. Start with 2 tablespoons arrowroot powder, then add in the mica powder. I suggest you add a little at a time to get the proper shade.

Mica powder can be purchased at many outlet stores online, so shop around to find the one you like the best.

Carefully mix the dry ingredients first, then finish with the oil. Make sure all is mixed and that there are no lumps.

When you add the oil, you are going to add only a couple of drops at a time… this is what will make the blush doesn't become wet. Mix well.

Have a mirror handy, and use a brush to apply a bit of the makeup to the apples of your cheeks. Keep a jar of makeup remover handy, and remove between tests.

Again, if you want a darker shade, try adding more mica powder. If you want lighter, add more arrowroot powder. It's going to be a lot of trial and error for your own particular skin type and preferences, but with a few test runs you'll get it.

Play around with the colors until you are happy with the look, and you are done! Store the powder in a small, airtight jar, and shake or mix before use.

Beach Hair Homemade Texturizer

What you will need:

Sea salt

Vitamin E oil

Purified water

Spray bottle

Essential oil in the scent of your choice

Directions:

Add 1 cup of water to your spray bottle. Add a few drops of the essential oil of your choice to the bottle, then add in the vitamin E oil.

Add ¼ cup sea salt to the water, and shake until the salt is dissolved as best you can.

When you are ready to use, shake, then spritz through your hair as you would any hair texturizer.

Homemade Dry Shampoo

What you will need:

Corn starch

Coco powder

White flour

Air tight container

Mixing bowl

Directions:

Start with your mixing bowl, and add in 1 cup corn starch. If you are blonde or have light hair, you are going to focus on white flour or whole wheat flour and corn starch.

If you are dark haired, try using cocoa powder or cinnamon.

Sprinkle the darker colors in with the corn starch, a little at a time until you get the shade of your choice. When you are happy with the powder, store in an airtight container.

To use, sprinkle some powder in your hair and work through with your fingers. Rough it through your hair as you would with any other dry shampoo, and style as usual.

Conclusion

There you have it, everything you need to know to make your own makeup, and to use the best ingredients to end up with exactly what you want, every time. When you are making your own makeup, you are in control of what you get.

Whether you are hoping for something that is all natural, something that is entirely organic, or something that you make yourself, you are going to get what you are after with this book.

I hope this book inspires you to take your makeup regimen to the next level. When you learn how to make your own makeup, the door is opened, and you are able to make anything and everything you can imagine. Let this book open the door to your creativity, and mix and match or modify the recipes to make your own.

There's so many things you can make yourself, and once you learn how to make things yourself, all you have to do is apply the techniques you have learned to make even more varieties. I hope this book inspires you to take your creativity to the next level, and make all the makeup you need from here on out.

The more you make, the easier it's going to become, and the more you will realize how you can use these skills to make more kinds of makeup. The more you learn how to make, the less you are going to need from the store, and the better your skin will look.

Your skin is a living organ, and it requires proper care to keep it healthy and strong. When you are using all natural and organic ingredients, you are doing the best thing you could possibly do for your skin… something that you will be so glad you did.

Many people use a variety of makeup daily, but they don't stop to realize they are doing more harm to their skin than good. Everything you put on your skin is absorbed, so you need to be mindful of exactly what you are putting on yourself.

With the makeup in this book, you can rest assured you are making the best choice possible for your skin. Look younger, feel better, and fall in love with the makeup you create.

The possibilities are endless, so let your imagination run wild!

FREE Bonus Reminder

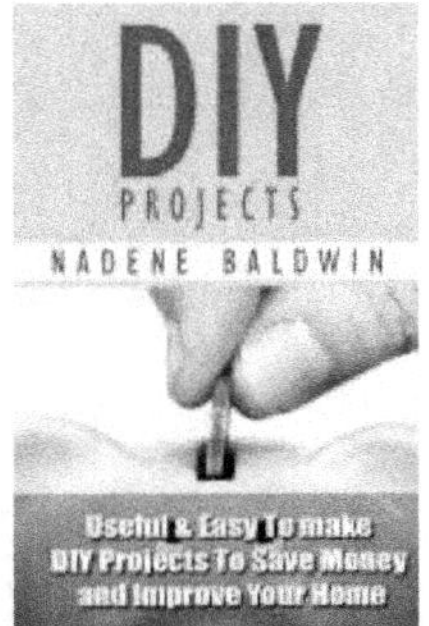

If you have not grabbed it yet, please go ahead and download your special bonus report *"DIY Projects. 13 Useful & Easy To Make DIY Projects To Save Money & Improve Your Home!"*

Simply Click the Button Below

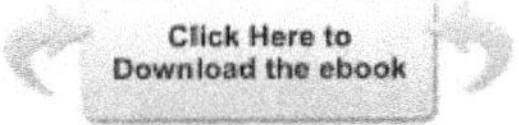

OR **Go to This Page**

http://diyhomecraft.com/free

BONUS #2: More Free & Discounted Books or Products

Do you want to receive more Free/Discounted Books or Products?

We have a mailing list where we send out our new Books or Products when they go free or with a discount on Amazon. Click on the link below to sign up for Free & Discount Book & Product Promotions.

=> Sign Up for Free & Discount Book & Product Promotions <=

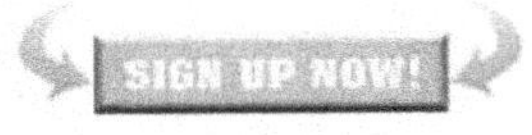

OR Go to this URL

http://zbit.ly/1WBb1Ek